I0104814

Half The Sight, But All The Vision:

Dawn's New World

Written by Shancy Dawn

Illustrated by Quill

Quill & Ink Publishing 2025

Copyright © 2025 Quill & Ink Publishing LLC
All rights reserved.

No part of this publication may be
reproduced, distributed, or transmitted in
any form or by any means, including
photocopying, recording, or other
electronic or mechanical methods, without
the prior written permission of the
publisher, except in the case of brief
quotations used in reviews, academic
reference, or educational settings, as
permitted by applicable copyright law.

For permission requests, contact:
Quill & Ink Publishing LLC
P.O. Box 133 Franklin, IN 46131
www.quillninkpublishing.com

Written by Shancy Dawn
Illustrated by Quill

First Edition
Printed in the United States of America
ISBN: 978-1-969109-08-9

This book is dedicated to every child learning how to feel safe and confident in a body that now feels new or different.

To all the children who see the world with one eye—

Know you are not alone, and the world needs you exactly as you are.

And finally, to the families who walk beside them—holding hands through the fear, learning and adapting together, and answering questions with love all while discovering that courage grows through connection.

Dear Reader,

Dawn's New World is a gentle, heartfelt story about courage, change, and discovering that being different doesn't mean being alone.

Dawn is curious, playful, and brave—but after losing an eye, her world feels unfamiliar and scary. As she learns to live with a prosthetic eye, Dawn faces new routines, big emotions, and the fear of returning to school looking different. With the love of her family, the kindness of friends, and the strength she didn't know she had, Dawn begins to understand something important:

Your eye does not define you.

Written from real-life experience, this comforting story helps children navigate medical differences, self-acceptance, and empathy—while reminding every reader that they are already enough, just as they are.

Perfect for families, classrooms, and anyone learning that courage can grow:

Even when life changes.

Half The Sight, But All The Vision:

Dawn's New World

This is Dawn. She's curious, smart, and brave. Although she's living her best life, Dawn has been through something that not all kids go through. She loves to climb trees, play with her dog Max, and wear her favorite baseball cap backward.

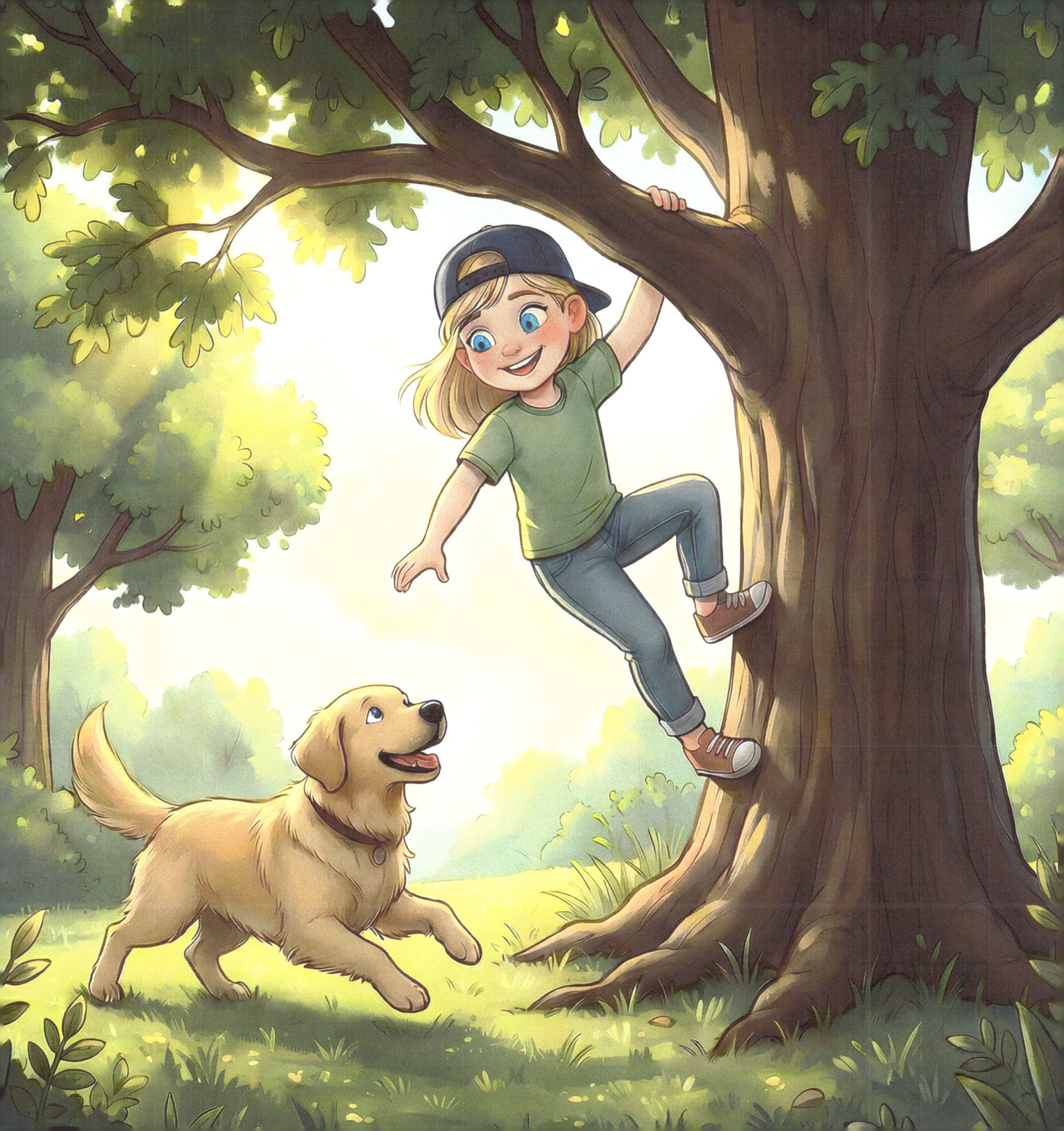

Something happened not too long ago that changed Dawn's life forever. One of her eyes had been hurt, and now it doesn't work like it used to. This new experience was very scary and confusing, but her family was there for her, which she needed more than ever.

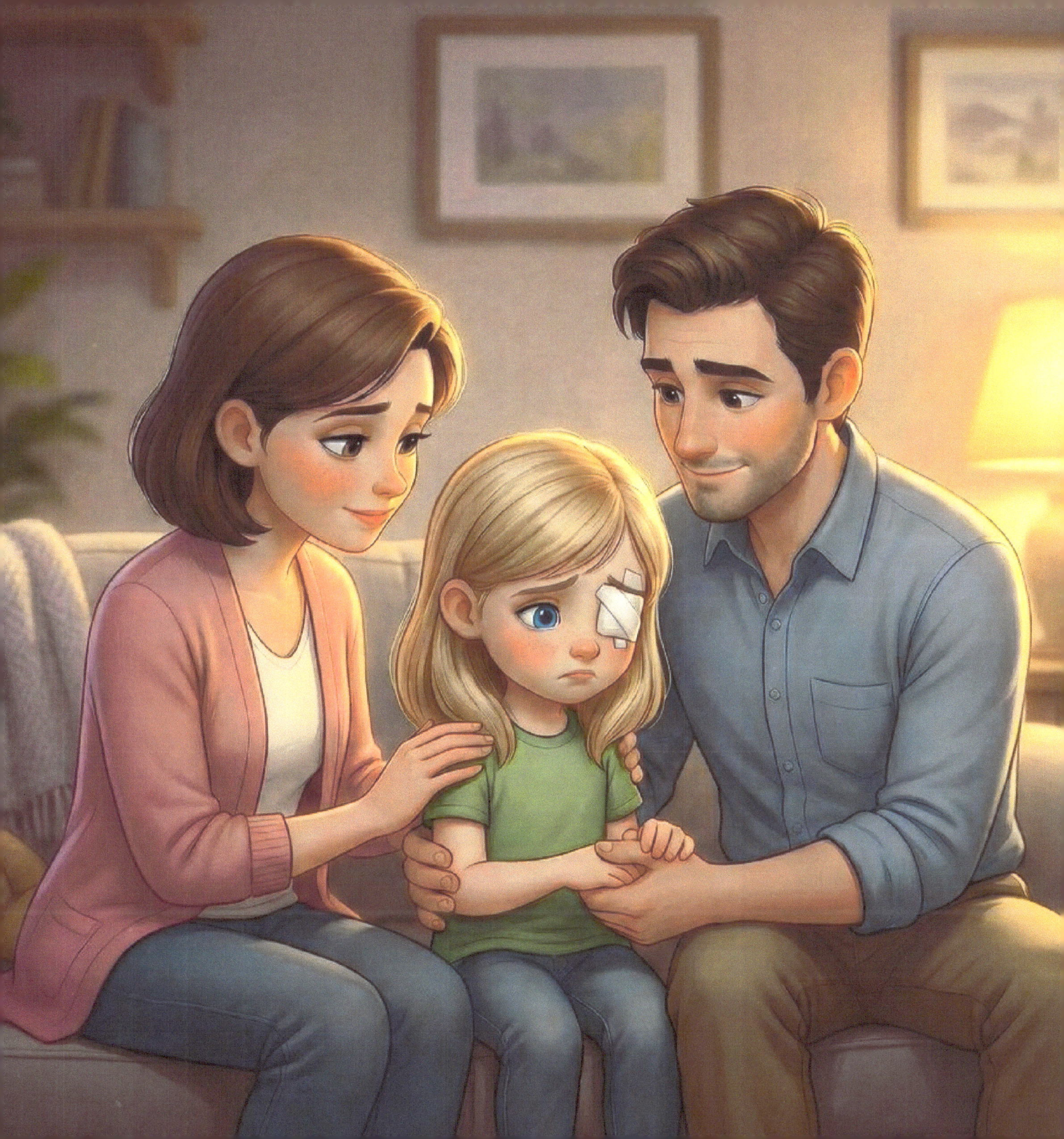

Doctors helped Dawn get ready for what would happen next: having her original eye taken out and then living with a prosthetic eye. It doesn't help her see, but it will help her feel like herself again.

Doctors helped with medical care and removed Dawn's actual eye. Her ocularist will provide Dawn her new prosthetic.

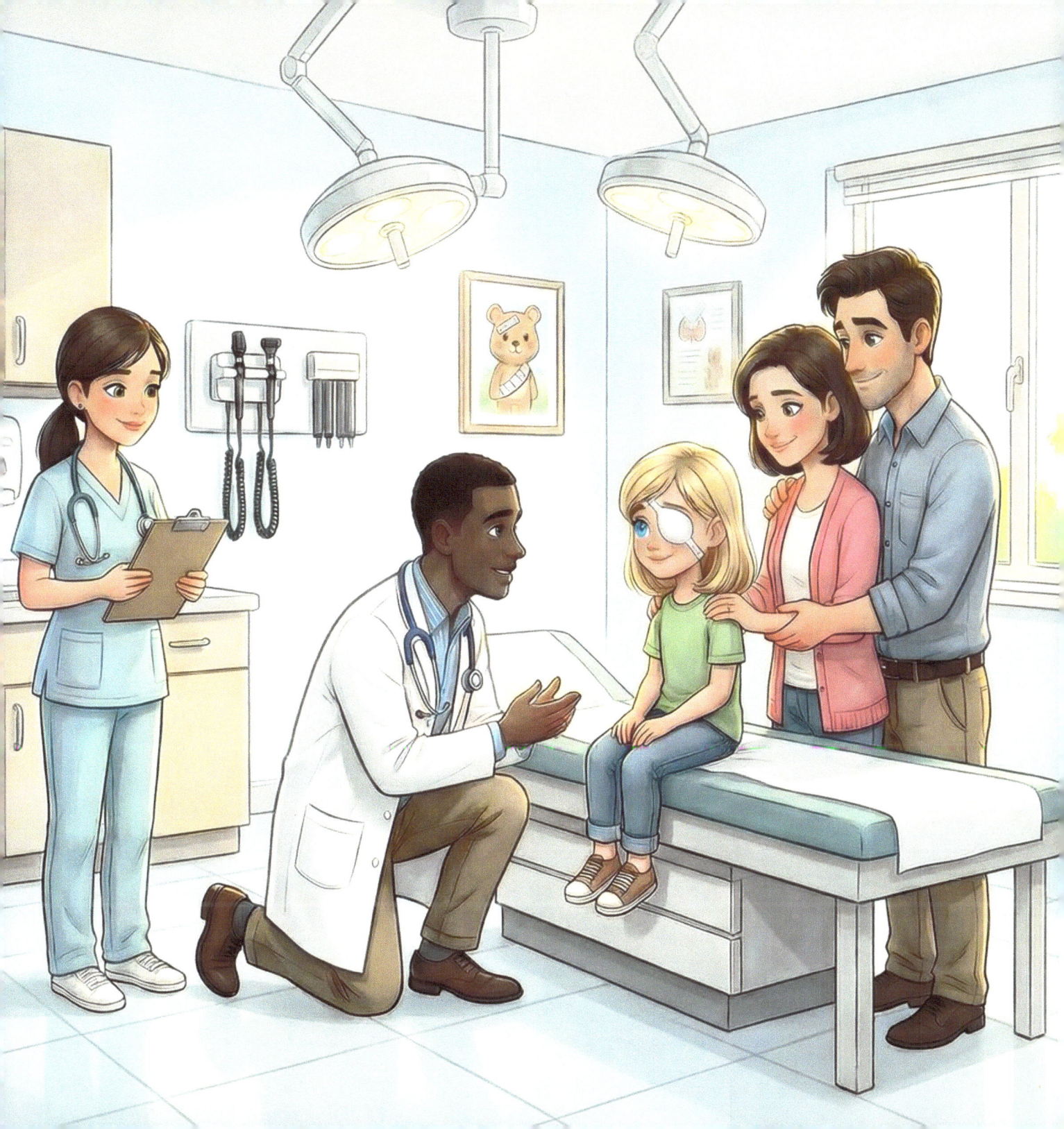

At first, it felt strange to see her own face. She had never seen her face with just one eye before. Dawn didn't know what to make of how her face looked now or the fact that her old eye was gone.

Her mom stayed close and told her that she would soon have her new eye. She also told her that even though things might feel different, they would get through it together.

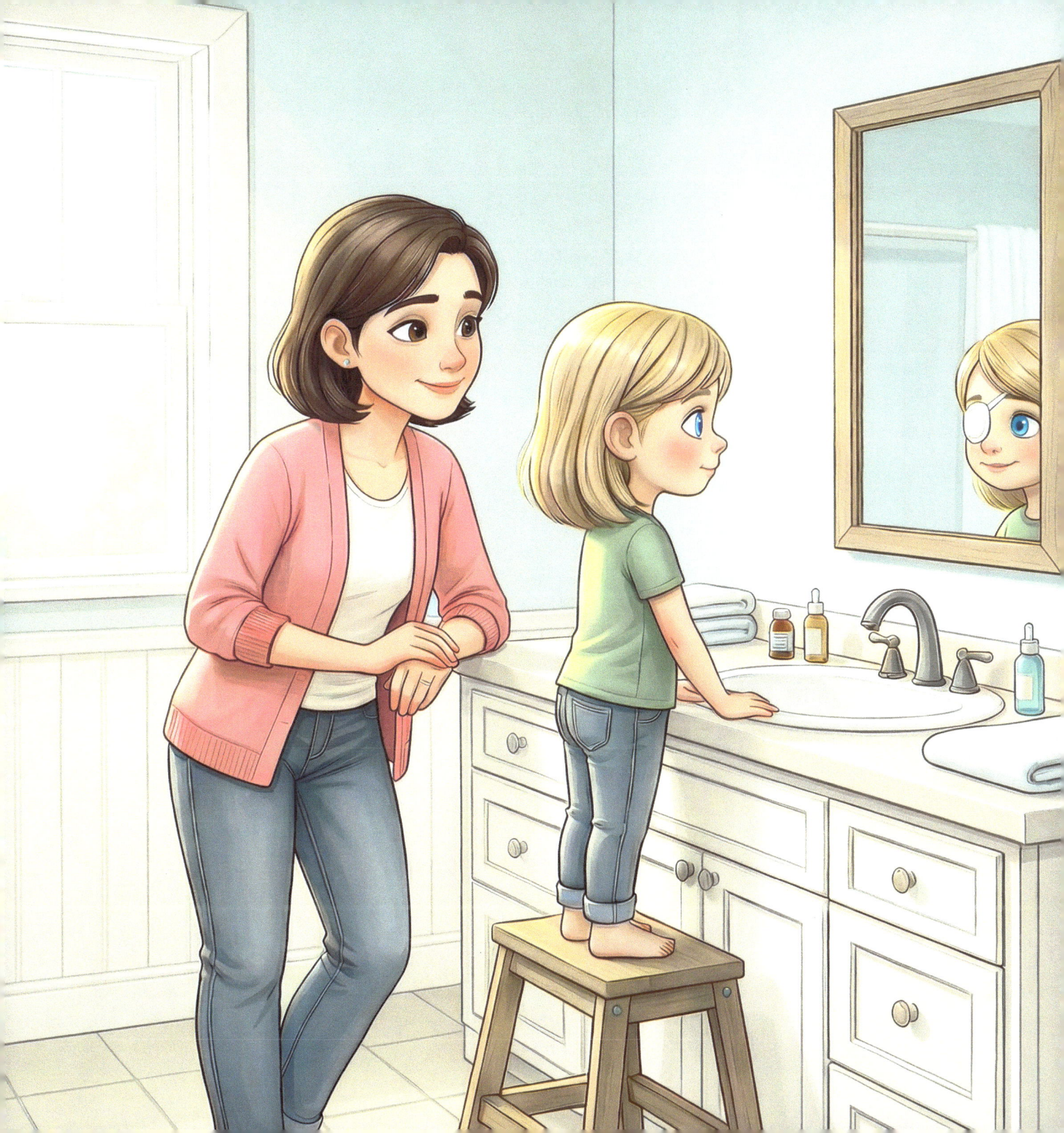

Dawn soon met Zach, her ocularist. She learned
that prosthetic eyes are both science and art and
that they are made to look like real eyes.

As Dawn looked around the room, she started to
notice photos on the walls—other kids, adults, and
families smiling back at her. She realized she
wasn't the only one with a story like this.

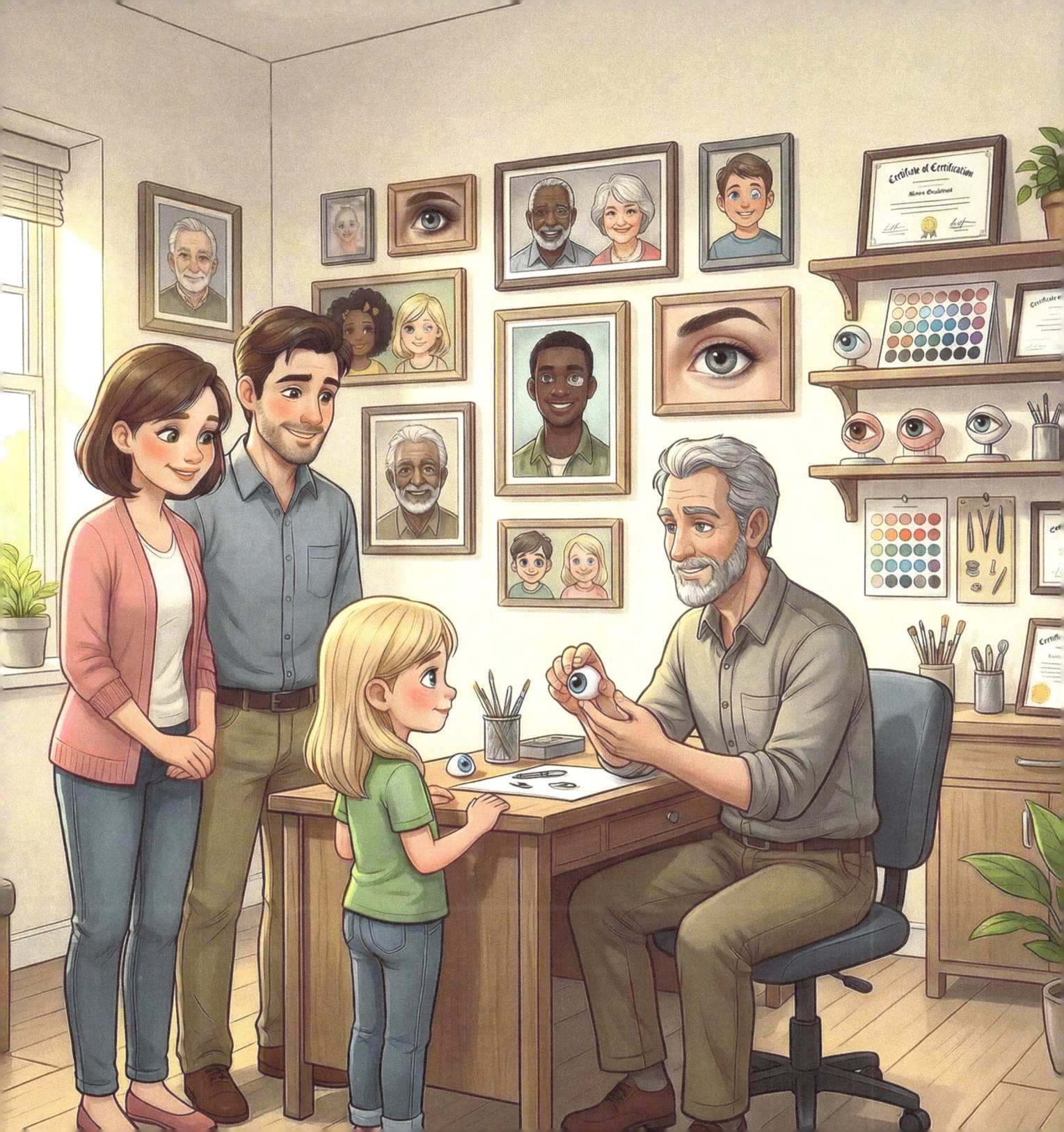

Dawn practiced her new routine at home. She learned how to take out, clean, and put back in her new prosthetic eye.

She also learned how to be brave and get over her fears when she touched her eye socket, the place where her old eyeball used to be.

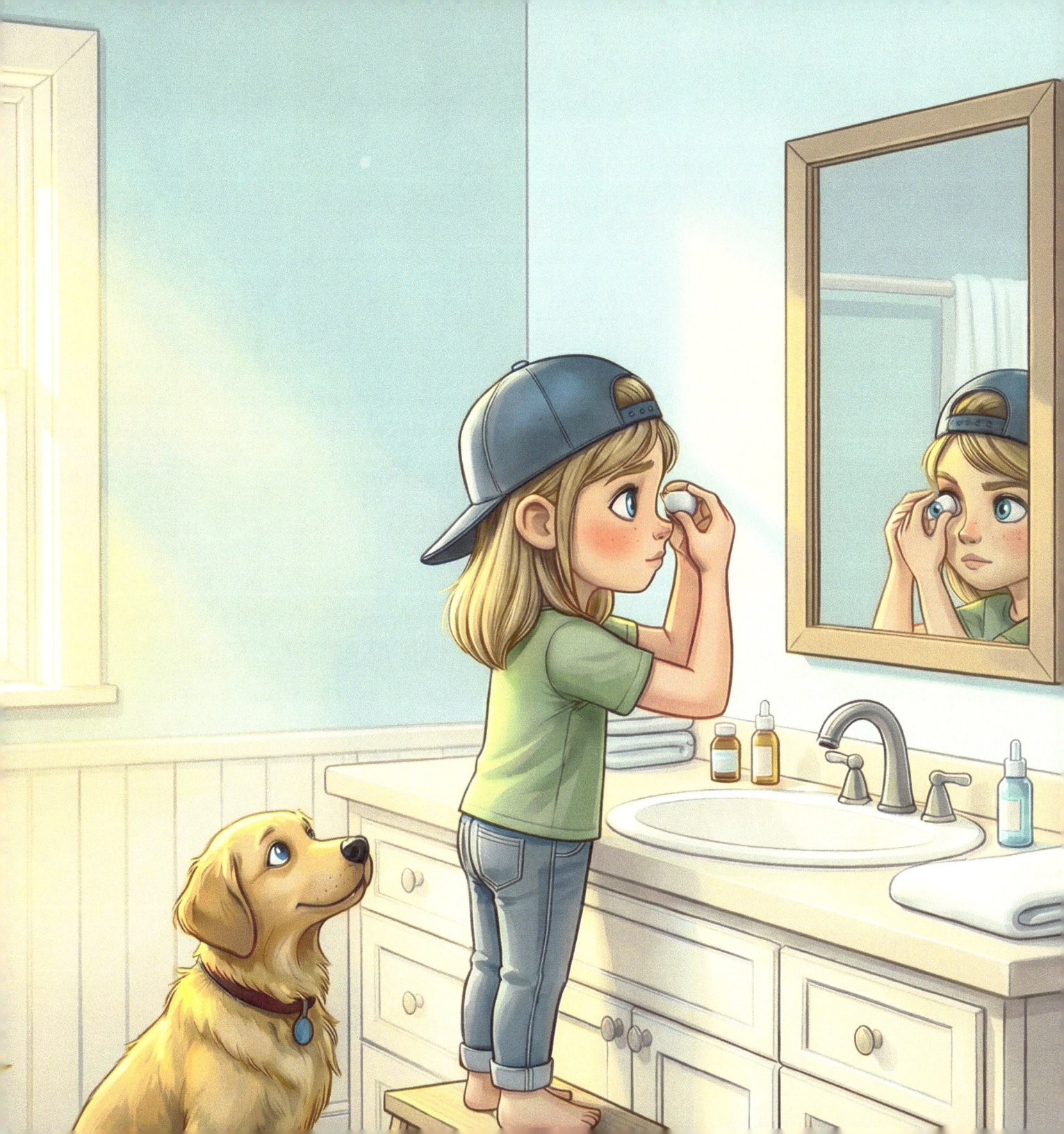

Dawn was scared to see her friends again. School had just started, and summer break was now over. She was afraid that she might look different now.

Her dad leaned in and hugged her. He said, "You are not just your eye; you are still Dawn, and your friends will agree." Dawn nodded, even though she wasn't sure yet.

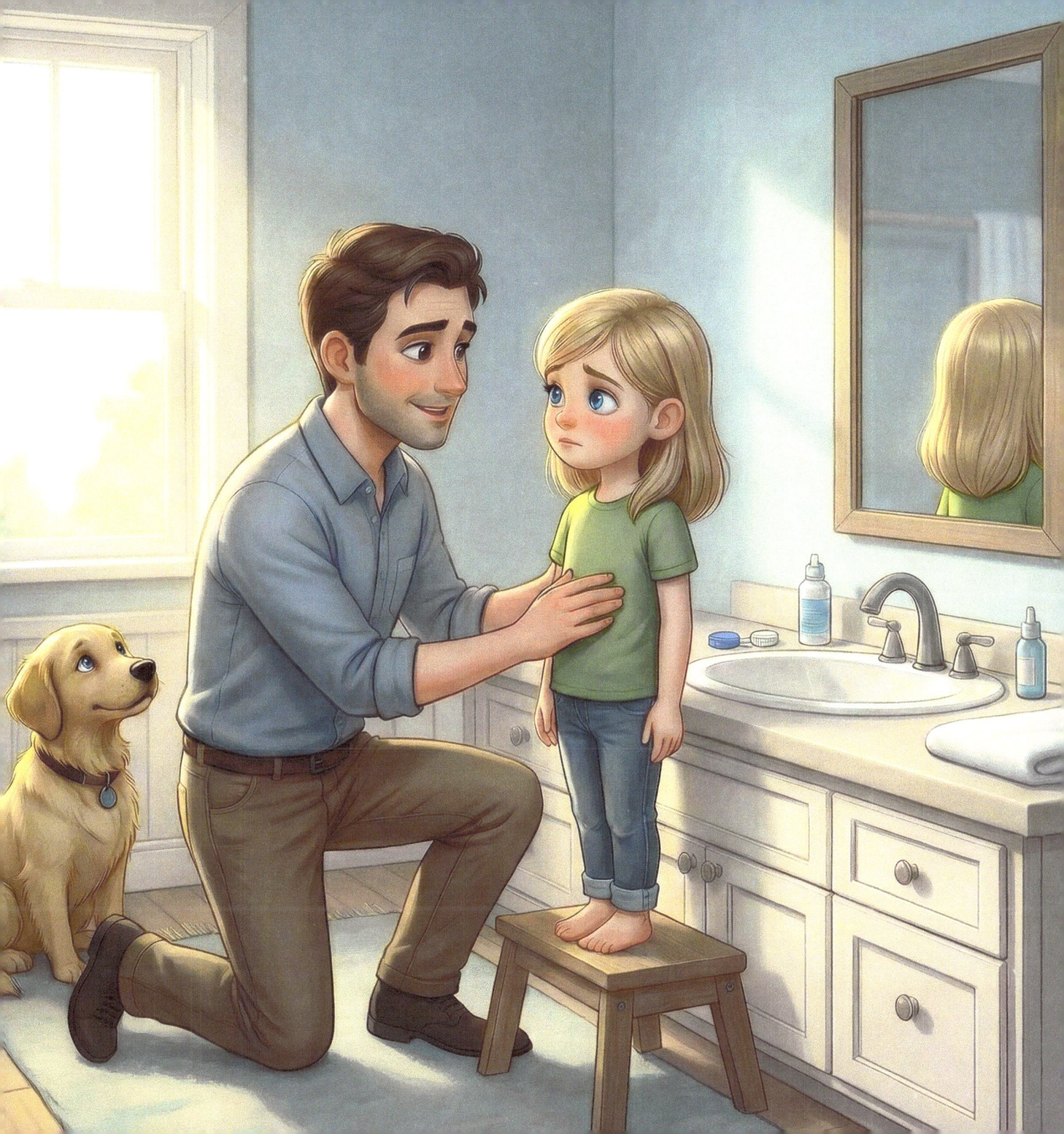

Dawn was nervous at school. She thought about whether or not anyone would see her eye. She tried to keep her eye closed even when it hurt, hoping she could get through the day.

However, someone did see.

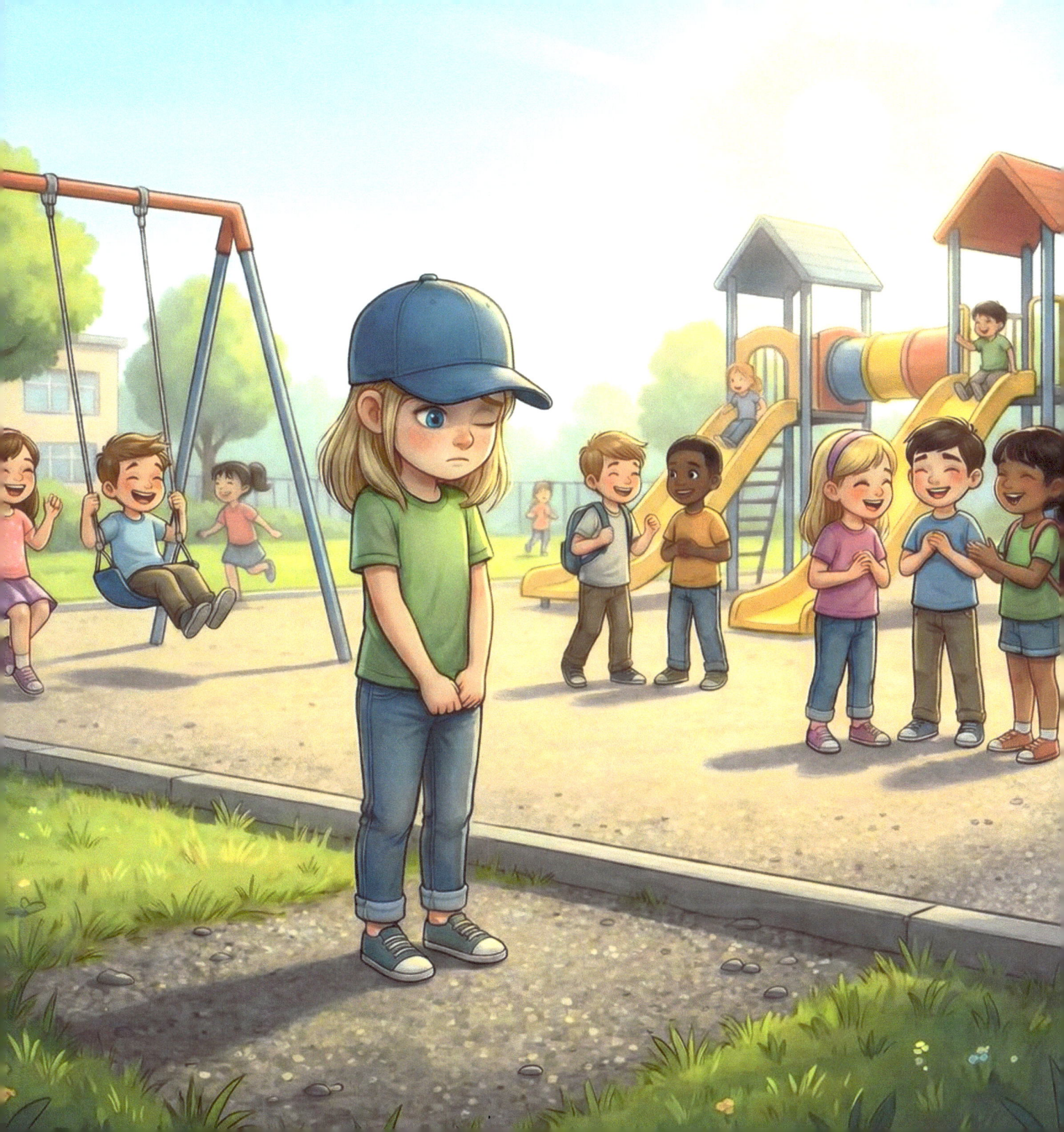

Her friend said, "Hey, Dawn!" "What did you do over the summer?" Dawn's heart sank, and time seemed to pause.

He saw... She thought to herself.
Her cheeks were warm, and she froze in place.

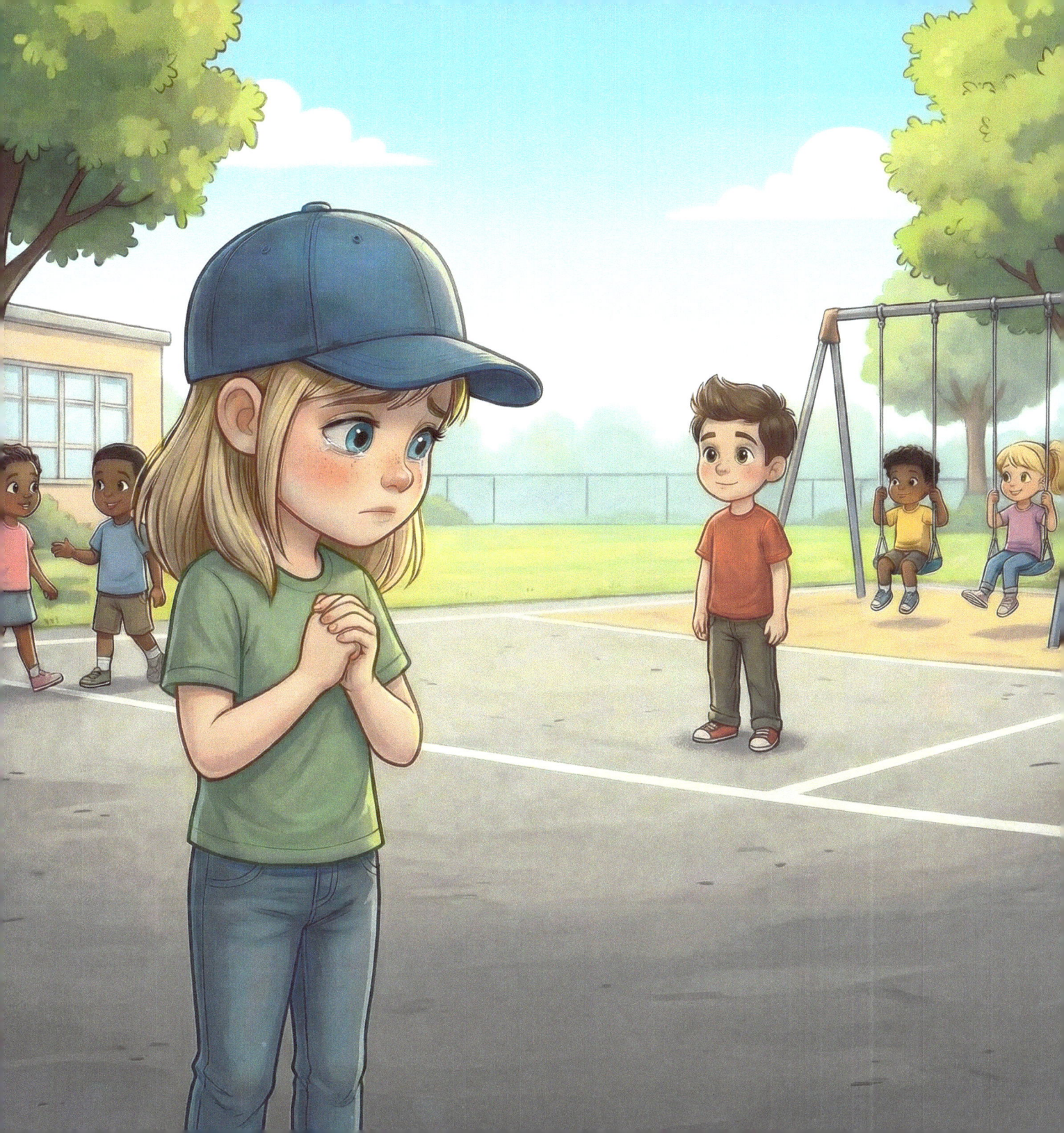

"Hi Dawn, Are you ok?"

Her friend asked as he leaned in.

She replied. "I lost my eye this summer, and I am afraid I look different."

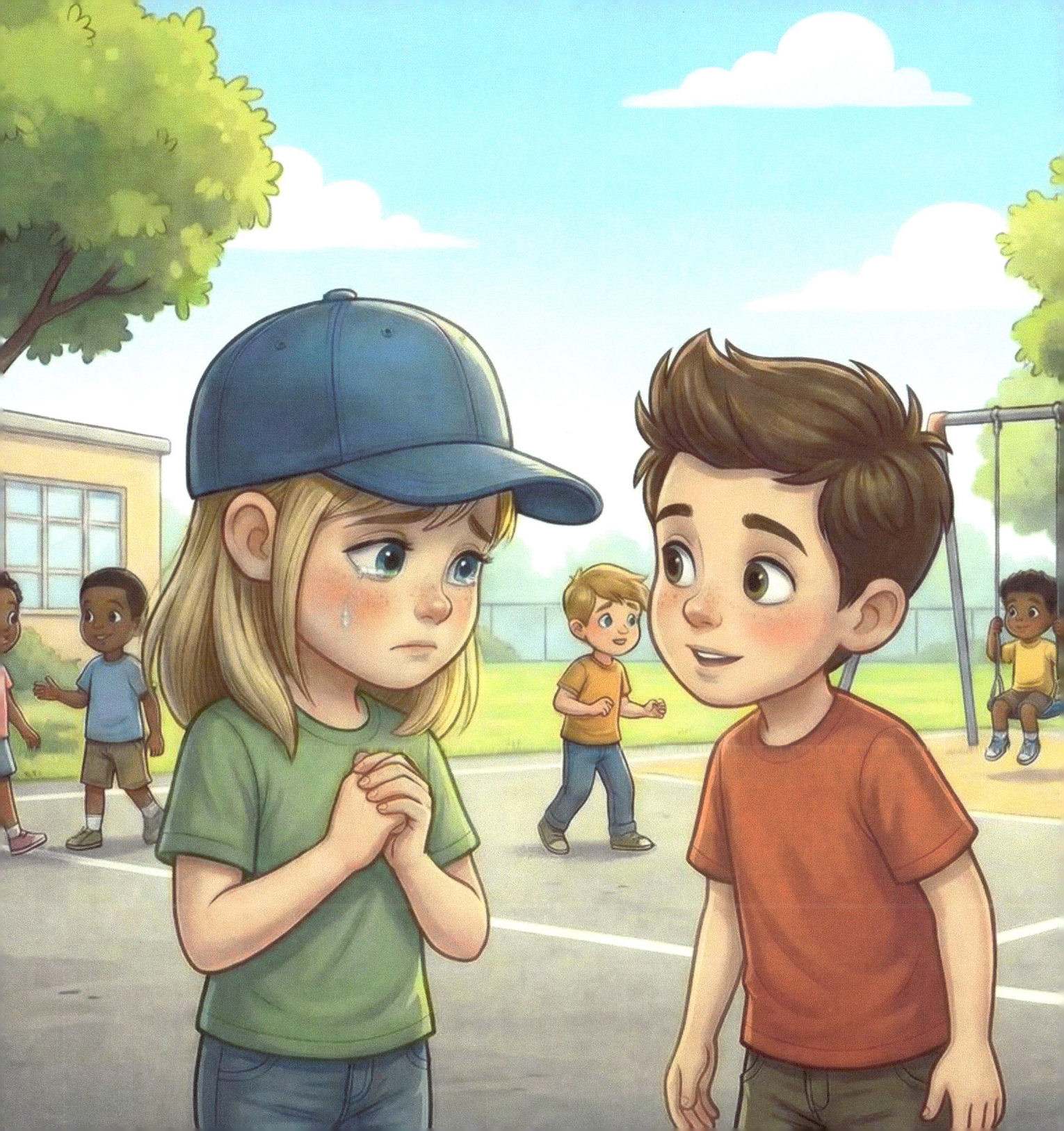

"You look the same to me," her friend said.

In that moment, Dawn realized that she was the same and her dad was right. Her eye does not define her. Instantly her fear started to leave, and she started to smile.

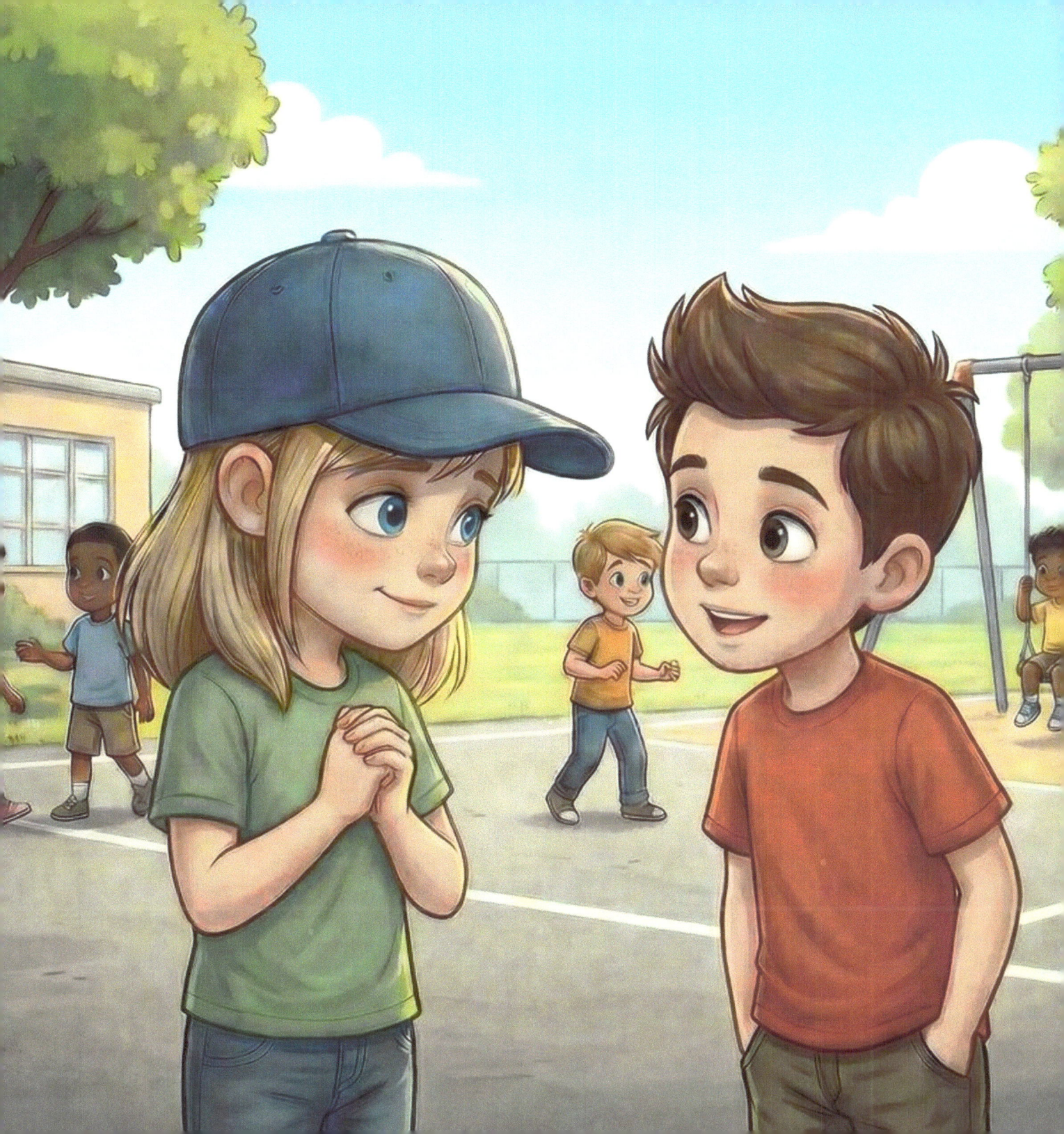

Dawn saw another student sitting near the slide as she walked to the other side of the playground. Recess was almost over.

Dawn walked over and sat next to her because she looked sad. Dawn asked, "How was your summer?"

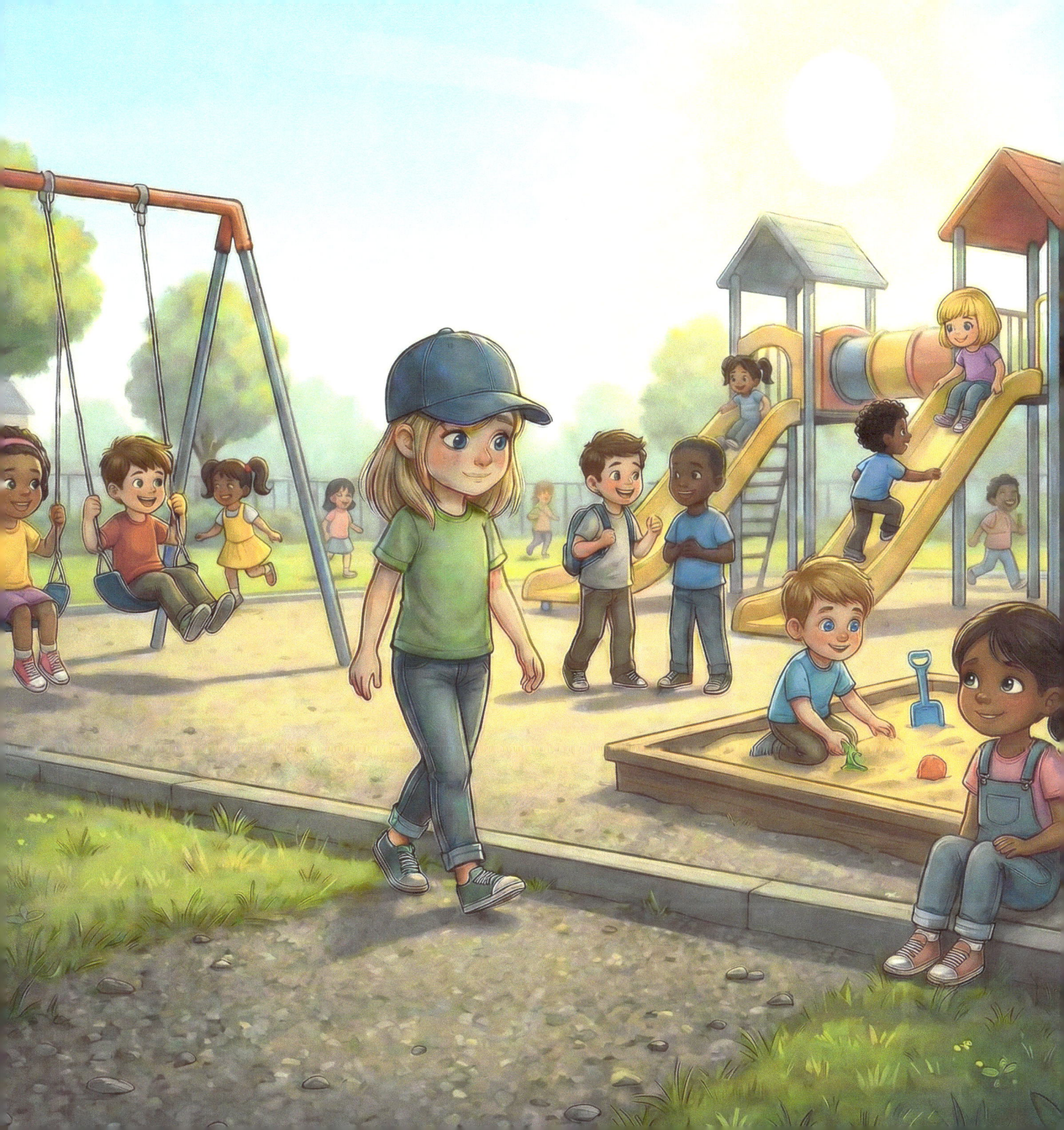

"I just started school and haven't made any new friends yet." "I used to slide down the slide with my best friend, but she isn't here anymore." – she said.

Dawn grinned and said, "I'll slide with you." "My name is Dawn, and I want to be your friend!"

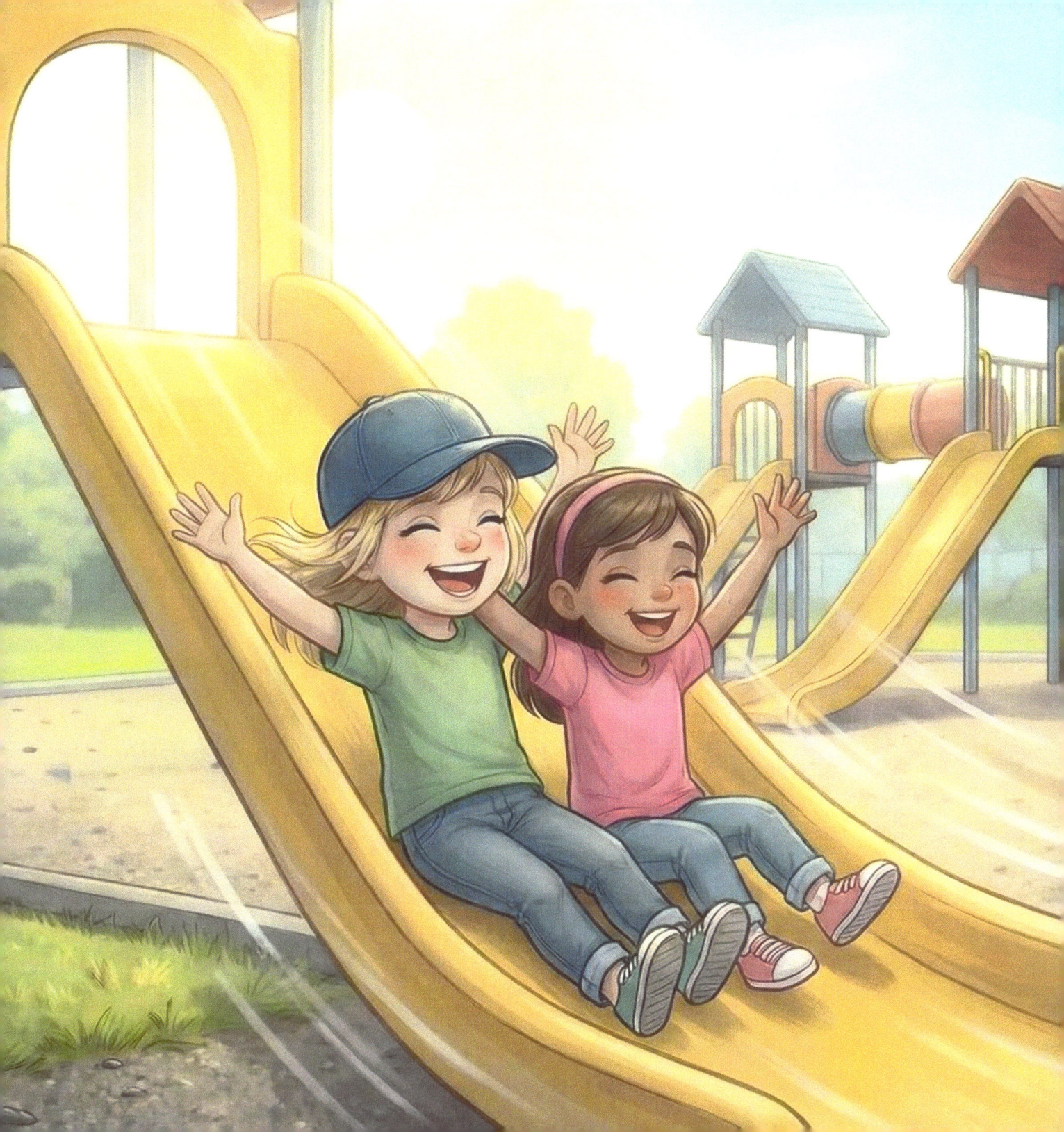

Dawn turned her cap back around at the end of the school day, just like she used to wear it. Nothing changed, and all of her friends still loved her. She even made a few new friends today.

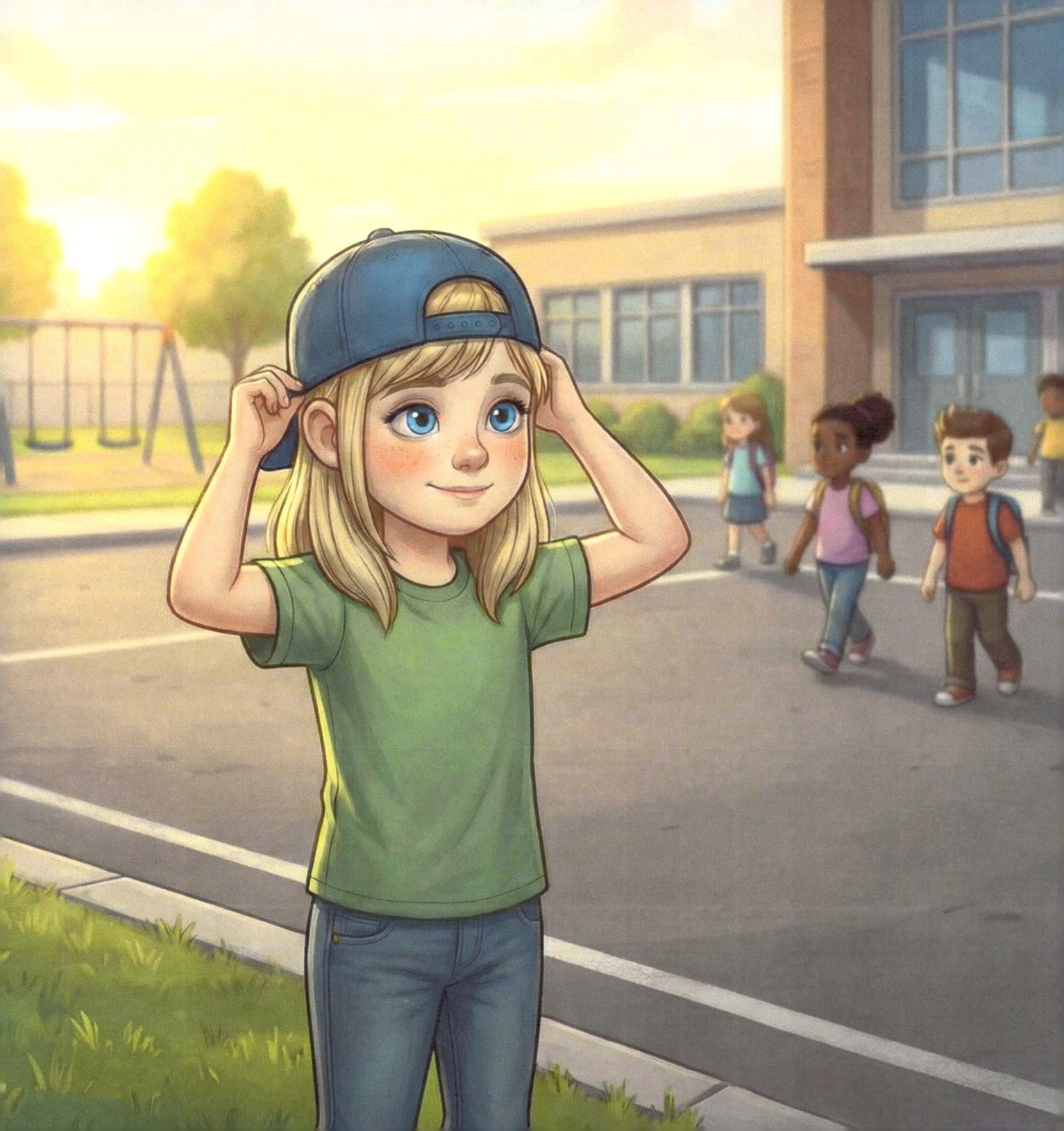

That night, Dawn lay in bed thinking about her day. Some moments were hard. Some moments surprised her. Most surprising of all was the way her friends acted.

It seemed as if nothing changed, and she was still herself even before her prosthetic eye.

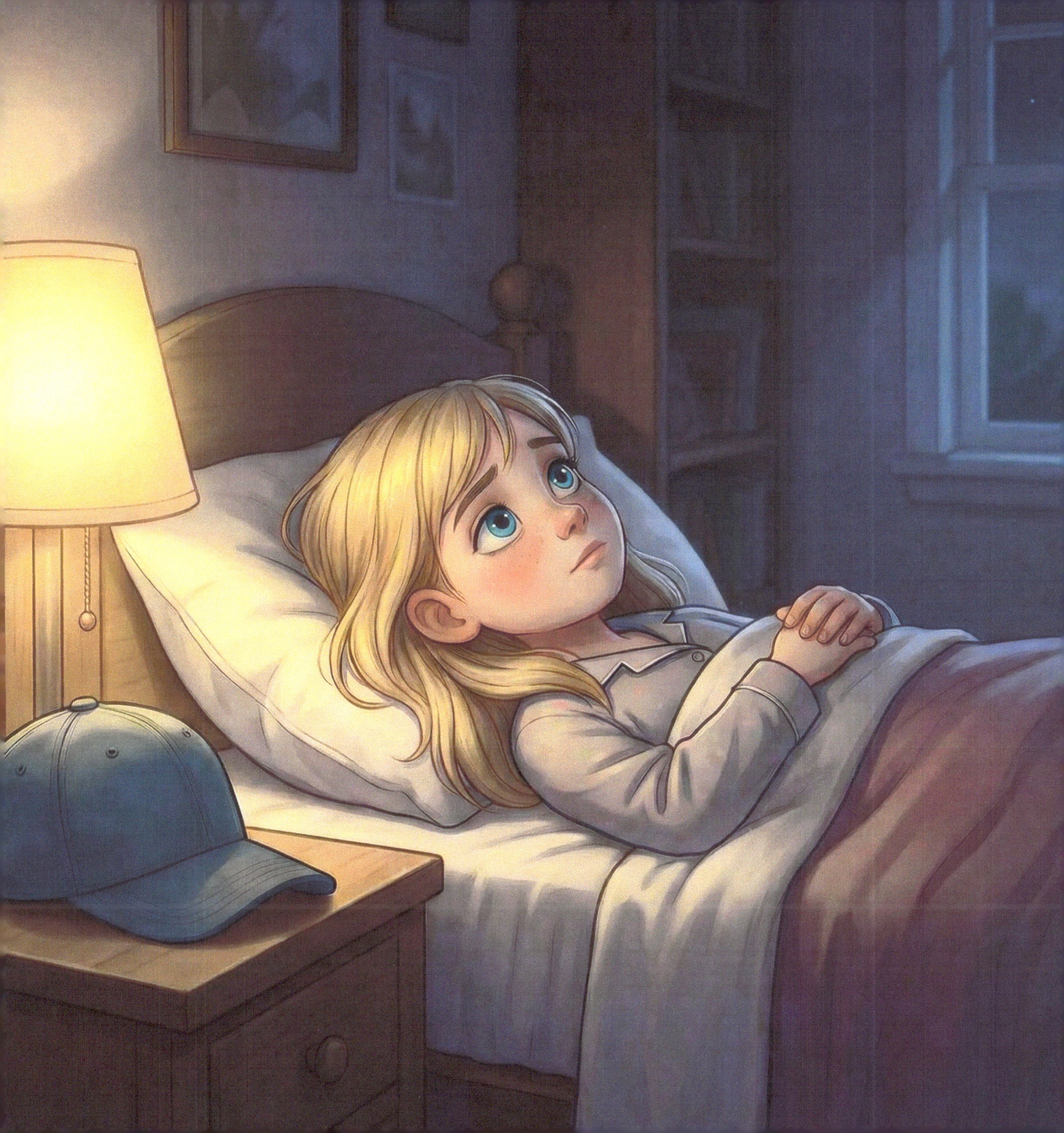

Dawn found out that being different didn't mean she had to be alone. If she didn't tell her friends, they wouldn't have known anything had changed over the summer. Even though she only had one eye, over time, she could still do anything she wanted.

People can only see what you show them. One eye didn't define Dawn, and neither does it have to define you.

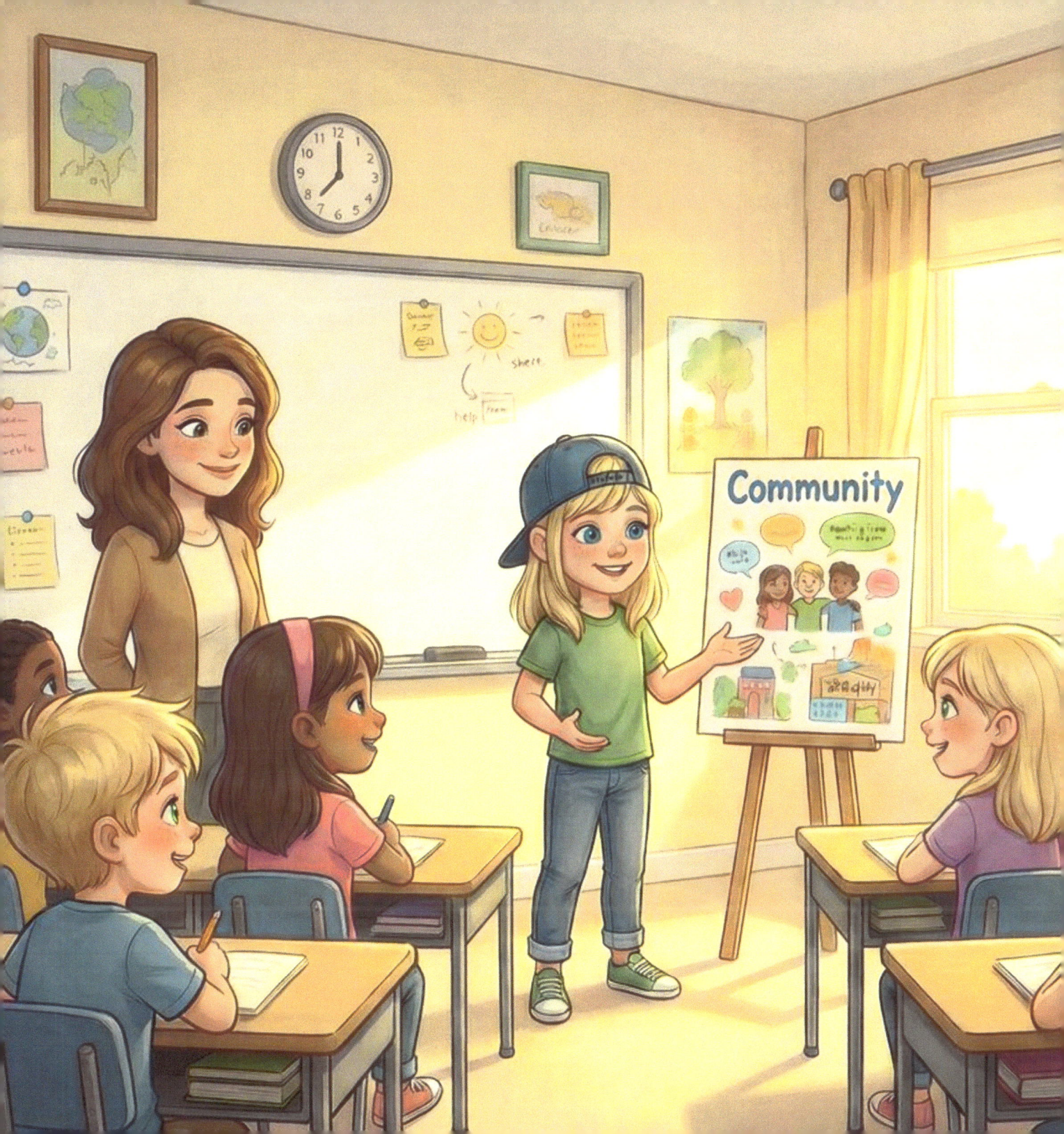

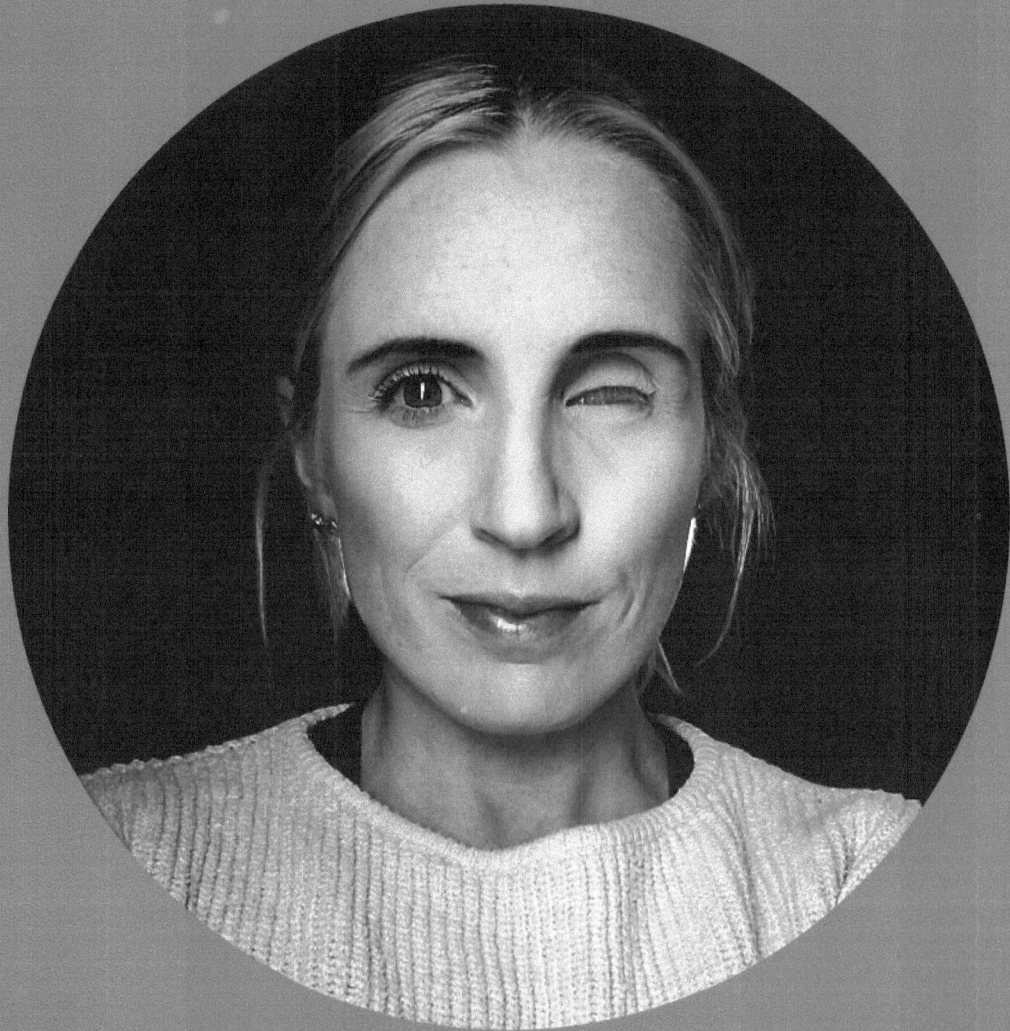

About the Author

This story is rooted in real experience—learning to heal through fear, uncertainty, and the courage it takes to adjust to life and body changes. Before losing her eye, Shancy Dawn had little understanding of what life is like for monocular individuals or how prosthetic eyes are made and cared for. Like many people, this was simply something she had never been exposed to.

Because most people never experience monocular life, this lack of awareness can sometimes make an already challenging journey feel isolating.

There are many reasons someone may lose an eye. Dawn's story represents just one path. Whether a child is born monocular, experiences illness, or faces injury, every journey is real and deserving of understanding and compassion.

Through this book, Shancy Dawn hopes to reach children who may be going through something similar and help them feel seen, accepted, and confident. Even when something major happens, it does not change who they are. Her hope is that this story helps children feel stronger—because they are not alone, and they are part of a community.

Connect with Quill

Shancy's story is one of many within our Real Life Experience Learning Series—
a collection of books inspired by real journeys, real challenges, and real growth.
If you or someone you love has a story that could help children feel seen,
understood, and less alone, we'd love to hear from you. Our mission is to turn
meaningful life experiences into stories that educate, connect, and inspire
young readers and their families.
Whether you're reaching out to share a kind word or explore the possibility of
creating a book together, we look forward to connecting.

Fan Mail & Letters

Quill & Ink Publishing
P.O. Box 133
Franklin, IN 46131

Email
info@quillninkpublishing.com

Website
www.quillninkpublishing.com

Follow & connect
Instagram: @ quillandinkpublishing

www.ingramcontent.com/pod-product-compliance
Lightning Source LLC
Chambersburg PA
CBHW060818270326
41930CB00002B/79